Birth in Blantyre
and the Malawian Birth Crisis

Written by
Alexandra Kulick

Photographs by
Edward Mikwamba

Copyright © 2018
Esther's House Publishing.

All rights reserved.
ISBN-13: 978-1985449947

ISBN-10: 1985449943

In memory of the lives lost too soon.

This photo was taken the day after your typical birth in America; a six and a half hour labor with an epidural and twenty minutes of pushing resulting in a healthy baby and mom.

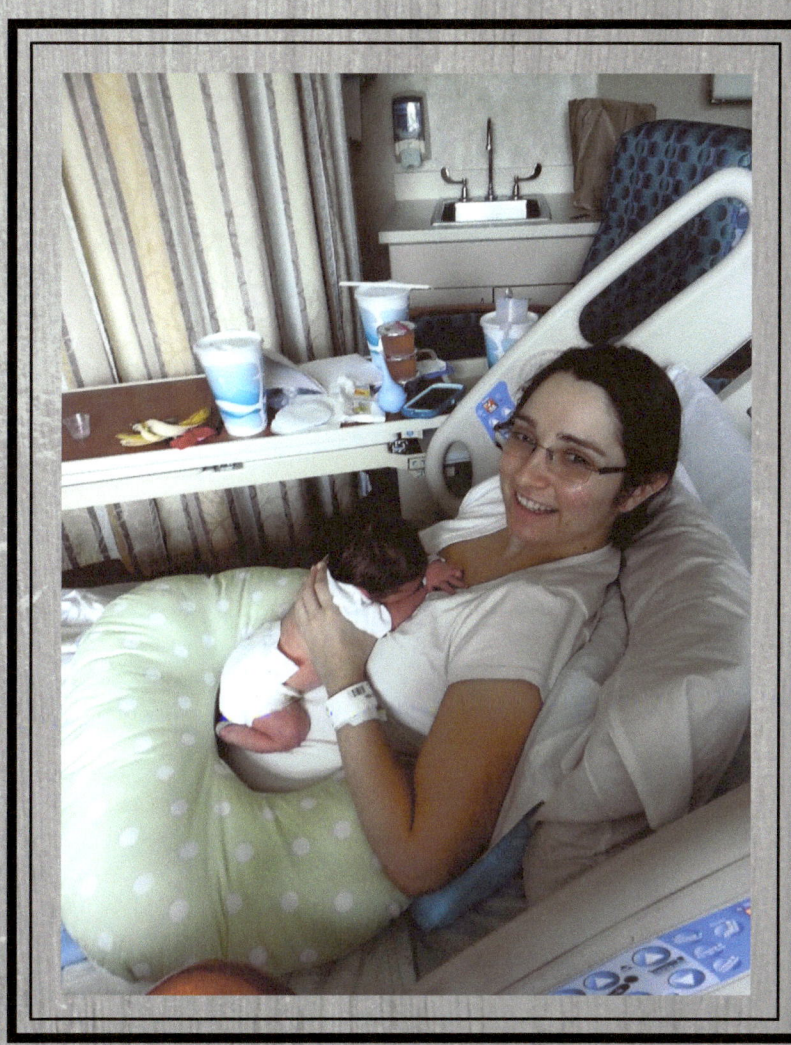

An endless supply of Jell-O and round the clock lactation support followed the birth, assisting the mom and baby with adjusting to their brand new adventure.

This is birth in America.

This photo was taken after a birth halfway across the world in Blantyre, Malawi. A beautiful baby and healthy mom experienced a quick and uncomplicated labor and birth. The very same biological process with the very same outcome, except in far too many cases.

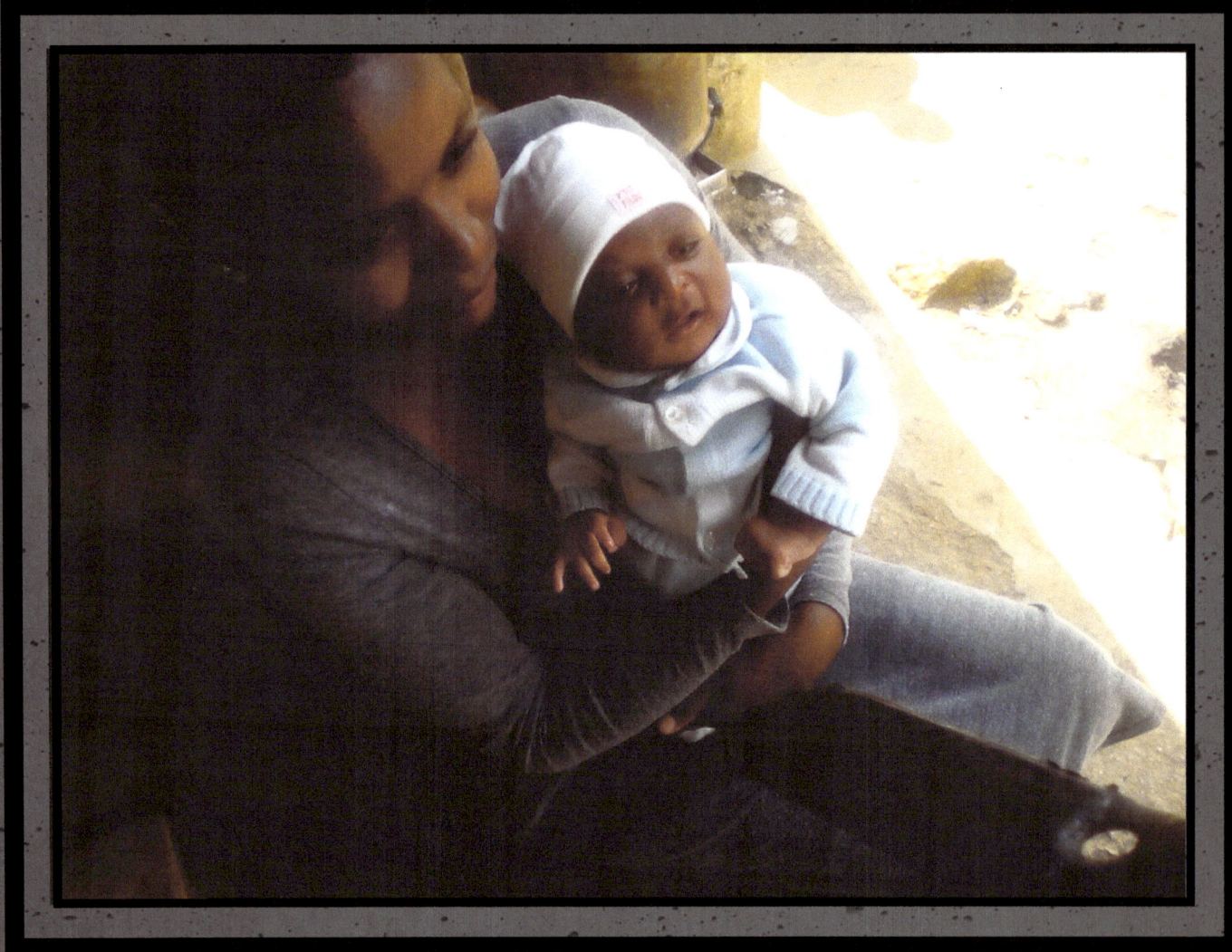

Martha M. Age 19

This is birth in Malawi.

Malawi is a landlocked country in southeastern Africa, surrounded by Mozambique, Tanzania, Zimbabwe, and Zambia. A country that is roughly the size of Pennsylvania is home to over 18 million people. Like many other developing countries, Malawi faces an array of challenges including 980,000 adults living with HIV and a staggeringly high unemployment rate.

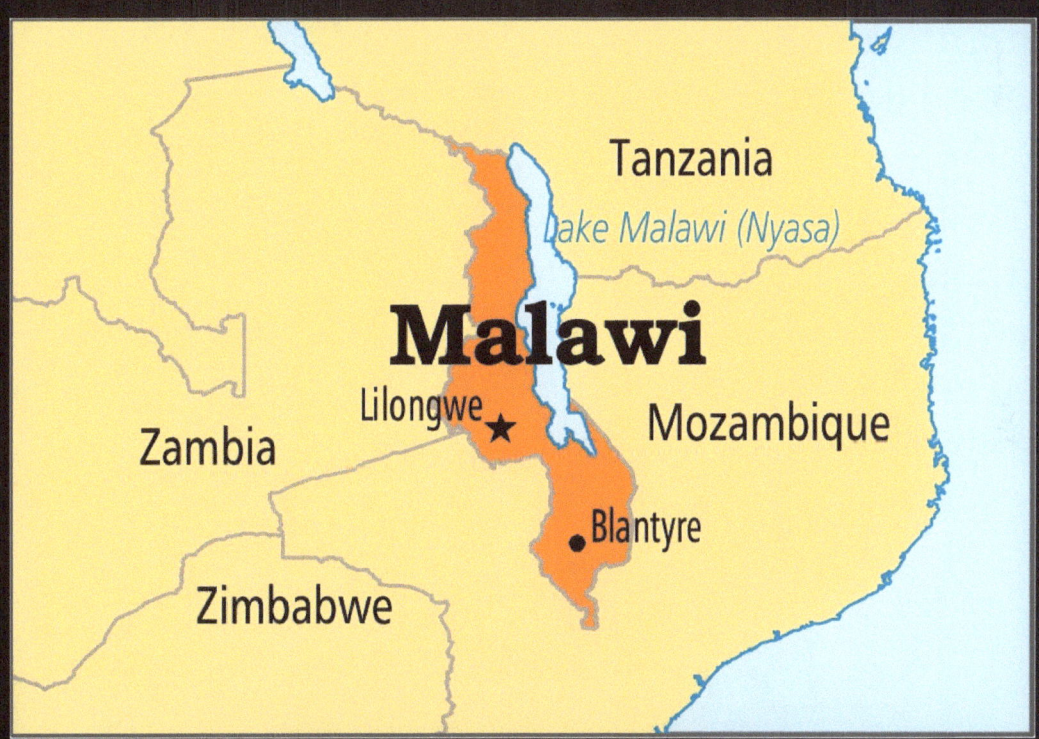

The Malawi Demographic and Health Survey revealed that 1 out of every 16 children will die before reaching their 5th birthday and 439 per 100,000 women die during pregnancy and birth. (Malawi Demographic and Health Survey 2015-16.)

On a worldwide basis, 830 women die each day from preventable causes related to pregnancy and childbirth (WHO, 2016). In my three births in America, the thought of dying and not being able to raise my children simply never crossed my mind.

When I started to learn about the struggles of a pregnant woman in Malawi, I wanted to do more to help, but first I had to understand the problem.

I had an array of questions about the birth practices in healthcare facilities. I envisioned babies being delivered by untrained assistants with out-dated procedures, so I jotted down a list of routine care questions and prepared to be shocked by the answers.

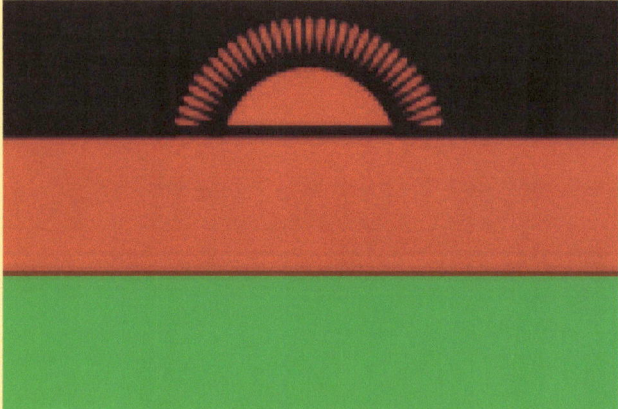

The Malawi Flag

The shock that I received wasn't nearly what I anticipated. An interview with Catherine Chande retired midwife, and nurse at Queen Elizabeth Hospital revealed that birth practices were incredibly similar to the care women receive in the United States.

Women are seen regularly for prenatal appointments, they're instructed about what is safe and unsafe during pregnancy and warning signs to look out for. Hospitals are even equipped to care for babies born before 36 weeks.

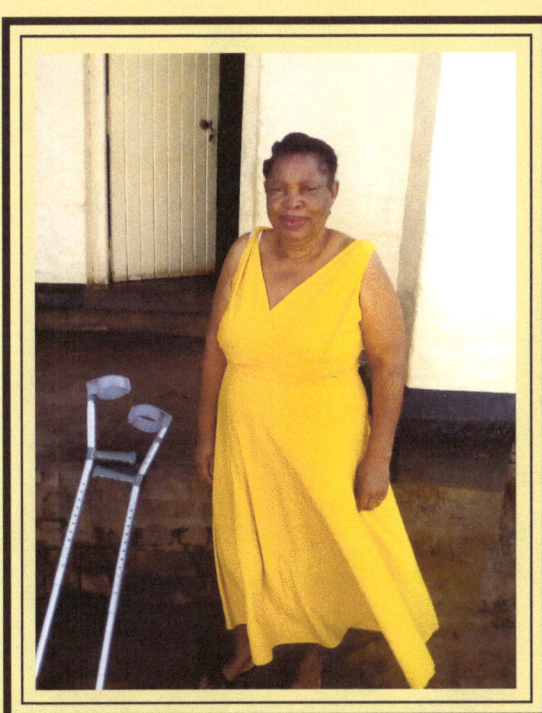
Catherine Chande

So, where does the story turn from routine care to deadly?

Catherine explained that in her experience, 3 nurses would care for roughly 40 patients per shift. The sheer magnitude of such a workload can easily lead to mistakes and complications being overlooked. Many United States hospitals strive to have 1 nurse for 2 laboring women and increase the staff if complications arise to ensure proper care.

Reducing nurse workloads can drastically improve the patient's outcome. One study found that changing a workload of 6 patients per nurse to less than 3 patients per shift would save 25 lives per 1,000 hospitalized patients (Kane et al., 2007). Increasing the number of nurses to care for the patients in Malawi could usher in drastic change, but it's not without hindrances.

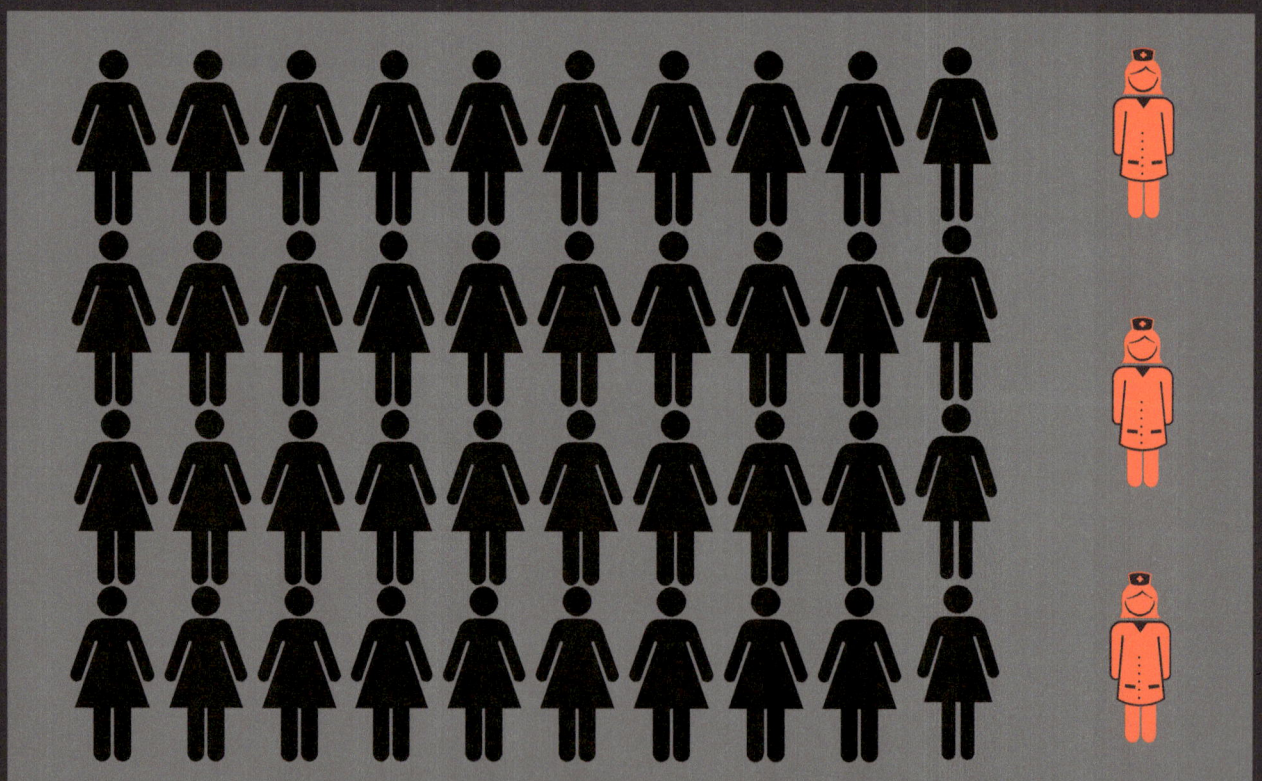

Becoming a nurse takes years of schooling and training. Though many may dream of joining the profession, the opportunity for an education seldom reaches those growing up in rural areas. Students who have the grades and money to pursue schooling are propelled by a passion which fuels them through an incredibly difficult work environment.

Hospital staff morale can be incredibly low with nurses overwhelmed by patients and working conditions. Nurse Jean, a beloved midwife, and registered nurse shared that laboring women were often shouted at for asking questions about their labor progress because the staff felt so much pressure.

Additionally, women seldom receive the instruction that they need to care for themselves and their babies after birth.

"Three girls verbalized staying [in the hospital] for four weeks because of non-healing wounds," said Nurse Jean. "There was no proper education on the care of episiotomies."

Nurses in Malawi face low wages, long hours, and little support, making this crucial profession daunting.

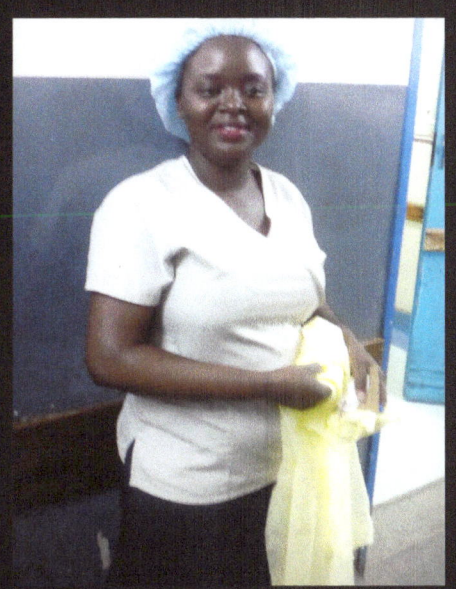

Traditional Nurse Attire, Nurse Princess

A New Mom's Reflection:

" I had two previous scars of C-Section so was somehow afraid of surviving the third one, but I got a baby boy and now I am joyed.

Hospital needs care! Our hospital are too dirty and lack proper cleaning hence one is prone to infections easily."

The shortage of staff can lead to delays in care, which can sadly turn fatal. In 2016, a comprehensive study was conducted to examine the causes of maternal deaths in a region called Mangochi, ninety-one miles away from Blantyre.

The study found that 96.8% women who died in the healthcare facilities had experienced delays in receiving care, and almost a quarter of the women died before receiving any care at all (Mgawadere, Unkels, Kazembe, & Broek 2017).

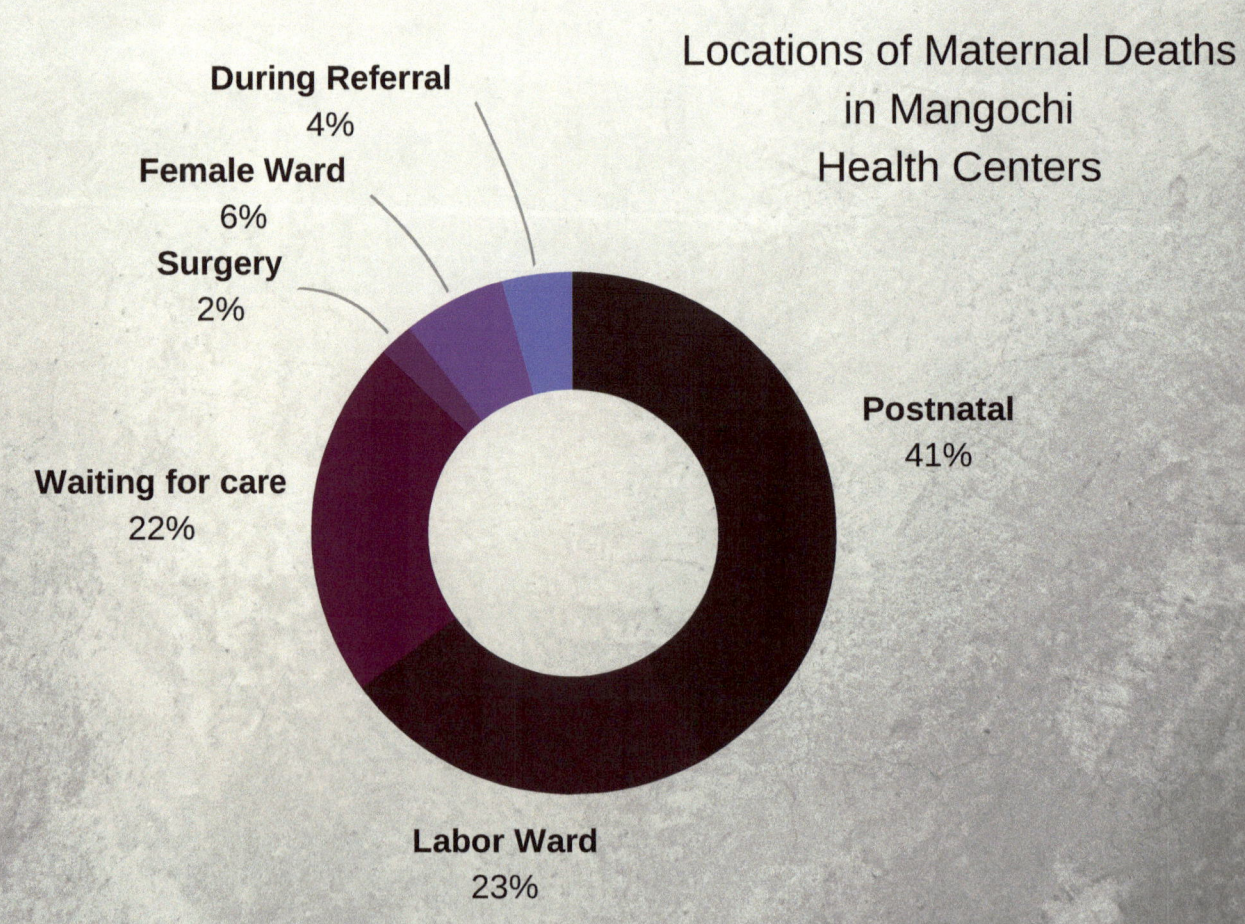

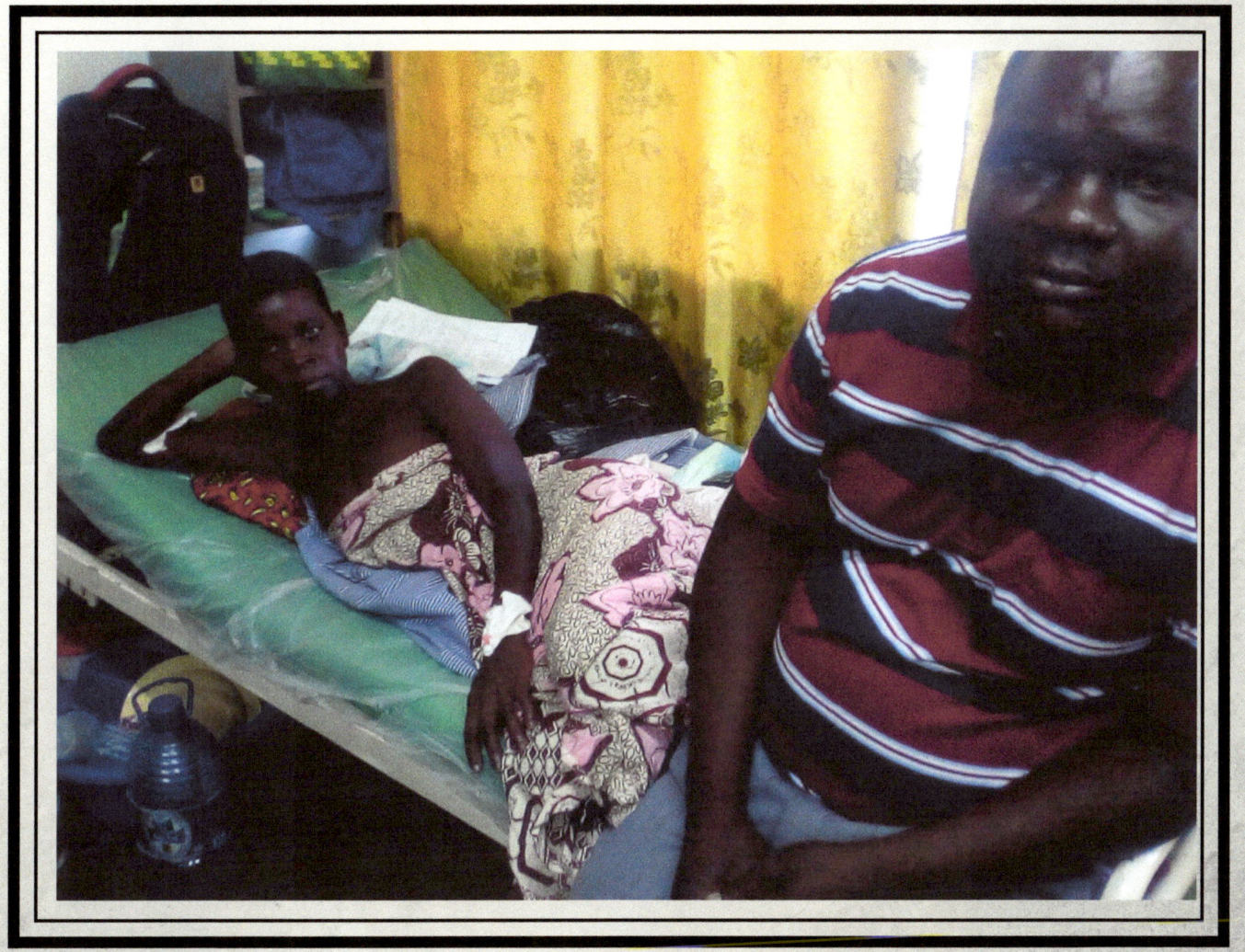

Rose Mutwana Awaits Care

Rose started having problems a few years ago after childbirth. The doctors suspect a tumor in her stomach or uterus. They removed part of her cervix for testing. While Rose stays in the hospital, she will share a large room with other men and woman, share a bathroom, and hopefully receive one or two meals a day depending on the food supply. Food and drink will likely be brought to her by her husband, Robert, a local pastor and driver at the Department for Health in Blantyre.

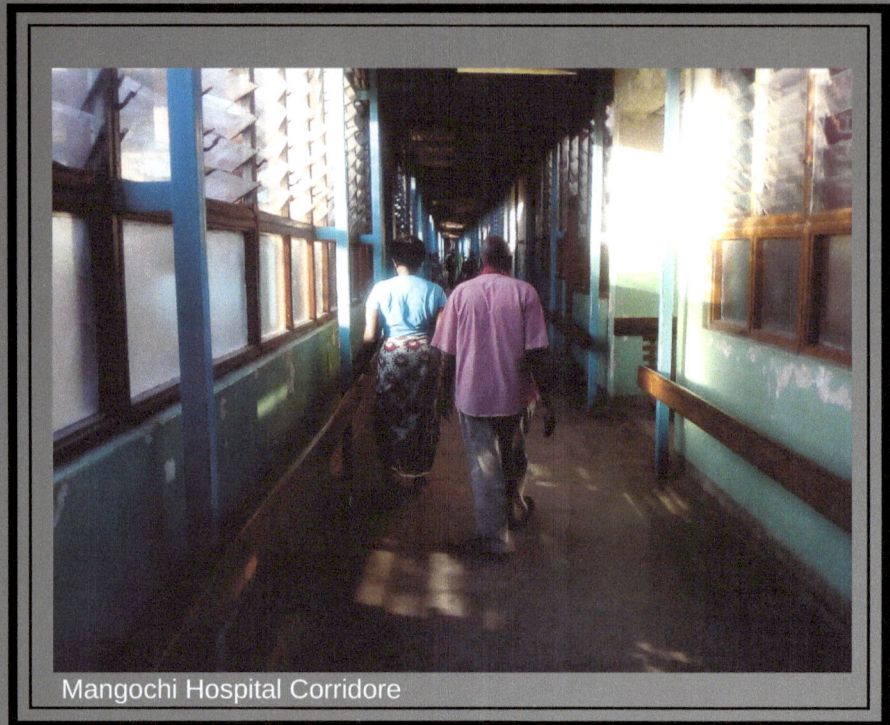
Mangochi Hospital Corridore

On top of limited staff, hospitals suffer from a severe lack of resources. Shortage of supplies factored into 63% of maternal deaths in Mangochi, including a lack of antibiotics, magnesium sulfate, and blood in the blood bank (Mgawadere, 2017).

BMC Pregnancy and Childbirth reports:

"Three facilities had an insufficient supply of gloves and healthcare providers reserved the gloves for assessing women in the second stage of labor only. As a result, seven women experienced prolonged labor which was not detected and subsequently died of sepsis."

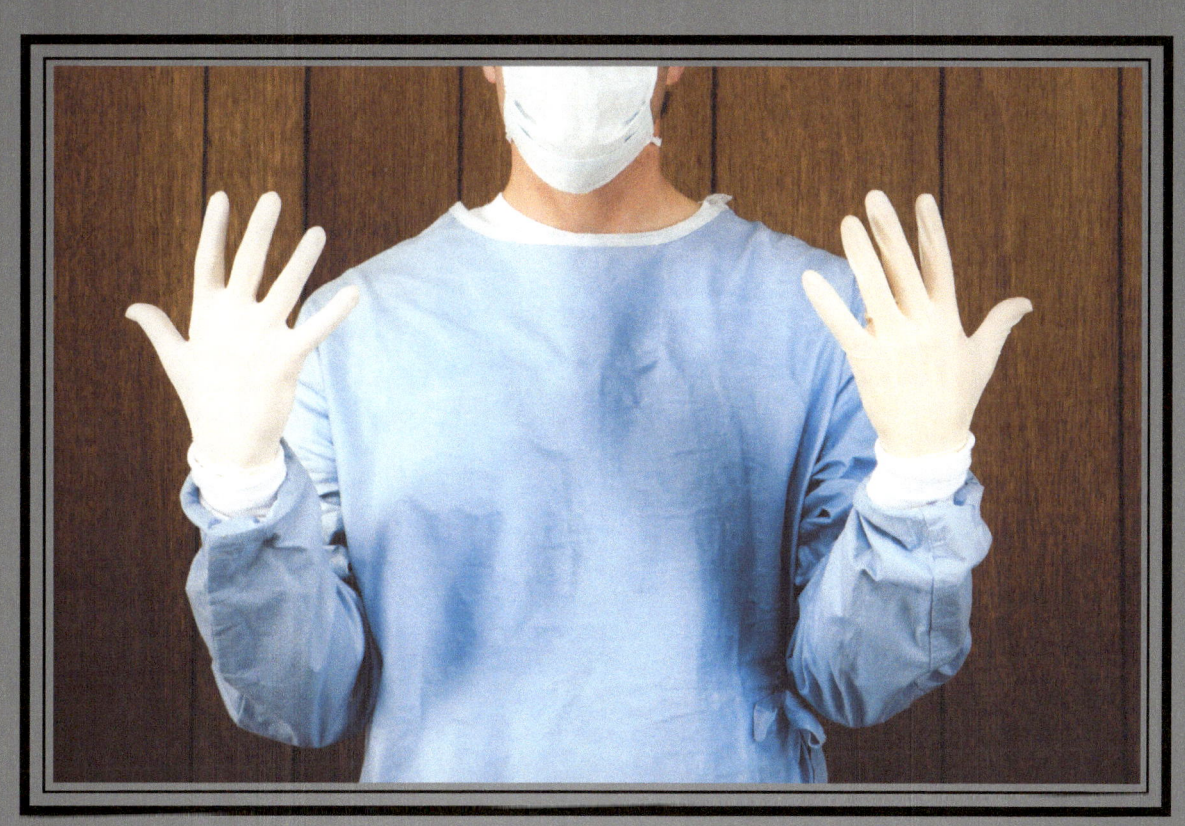

One box of 50 latex gloves can be purchased in Malawi for $6.
7 women died in one area because of a 12 cent pair of gloves.

I spent time speaking with Rosetta Swinton, a native of South Carolina. Rosetta studied nursing in the U.S. and sold all of her belongings to move to Malawi in 2008 and serve the community of Blantyre's needs.

Rosetta shared more stories about the developing healthcare system that seemed unimaginable.

"It is difficult to wrap your brain around," she said.

"I have volunteered for about 5 years because the staffing was always inadequate. When you think of hospitals at 100% capacity in the US, you can have hospitals here at 600%. A bed for 1 sick bay can contain 4, all sharing from the same one oxygen tank with spliced tubes going to each one."

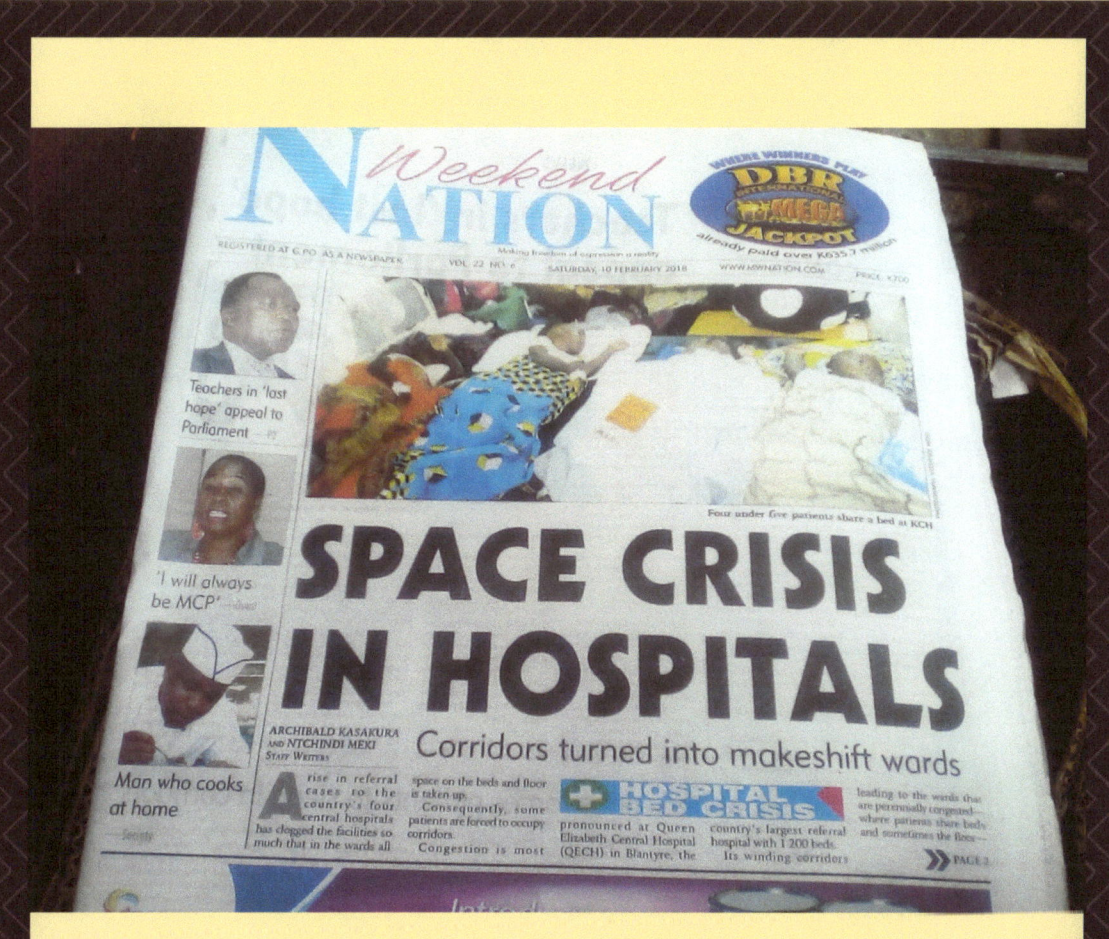

The Weekend Nation, a Malawian newspaper showing one bed occupied by four sick children (Meki 2018). Many have reported that beds can be made available for $100.

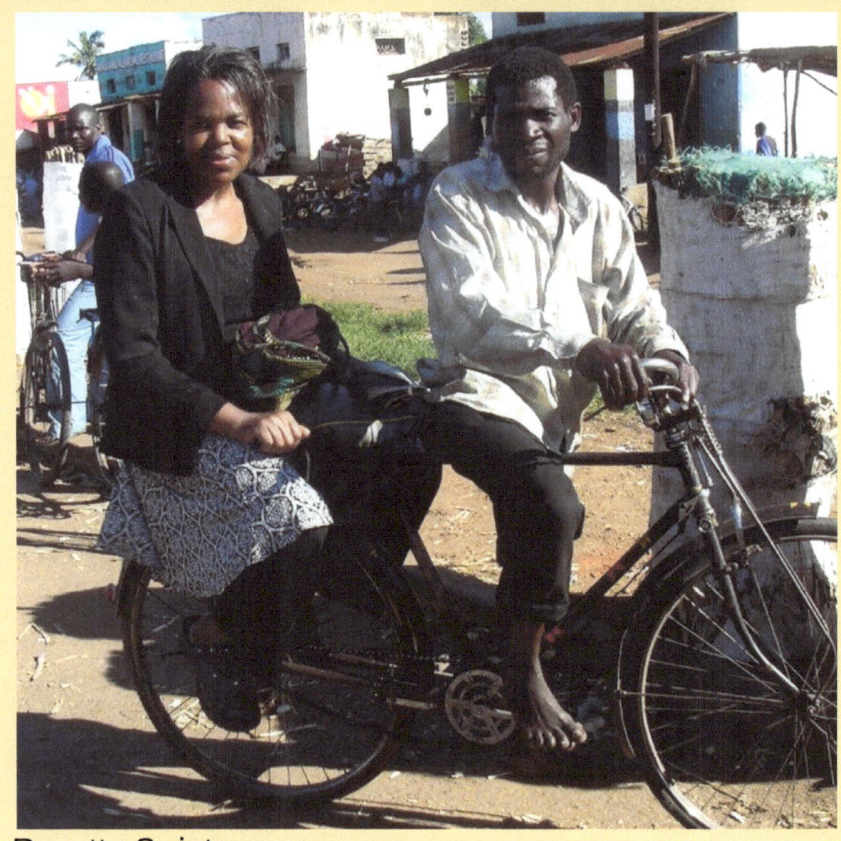
Rosetta Swinton

"We did a mission outreach in the capital at a government hospital where they did not have a functioning dental chair, people of all ages were lined up on queue for tooth extractions to have a perfectly good tooth that only needed a filling or tooth canal, but the basic supplies for fillings are never available....they do a local [anesthetic] and then pull!" explained Rosetta.

Rosetta also alerted me to another startling problem affecting countless lives: blackouts.

Imagine delivering a baby with the light from your cell phone because the power went out. That's the unexpected reality many health facilities face in the wake of Malawi's unstable power grid.

Dorothy Ngoma, Director of The National Organization of Nurses and Midwives, told the Nyasa Times that the country's healthcare is in crisis after the deaths of patients because of blackouts.

"There are people's lives concerned here," she said, adding, "we are witnessing the worst incident of a crumbling health service delivery system in recent times."

Speaking on Times Radio, Ngoma said: "We have cases of premature babies dying in hospitals due to the absence of power for the incubators and whenever authorities are told about these things, they would ask for names of those children who are dying. I say this is unacceptable."(Muheya 2017).

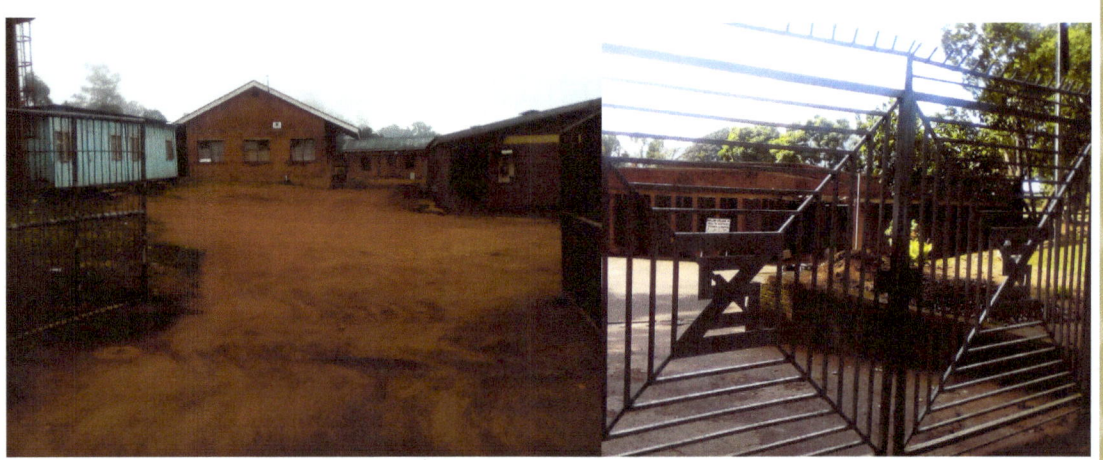
Limbe Health Center

Rosetta shared that often families would provide their own diesel fuel for backup generators if a loved one was having surgery, but generators were not always available. Sadly, the loss of power during many procedures can result in medical mistakes or the sudden death of the patient. Yet, that is a daily reality in Malawi.

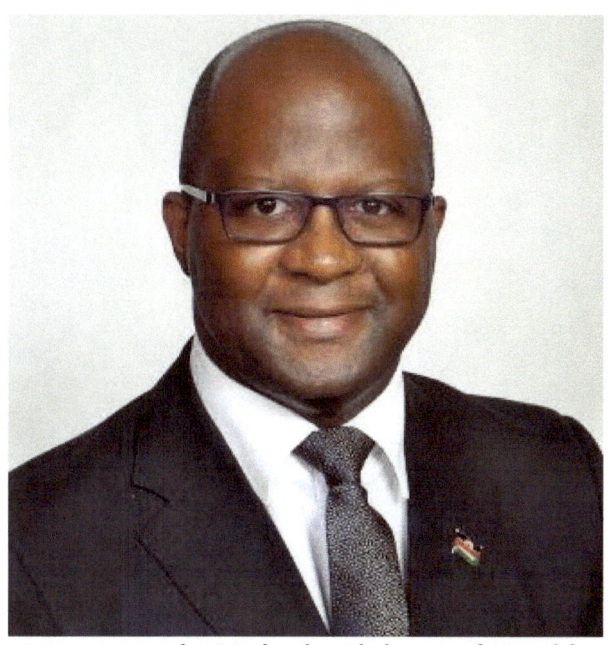
Hon Atupele Muluzi, Minister of Health

The Malawian government has started an initiative to outfit hospitals with solar panels to provide backup power. But for those whose lives are at the mercy of the power grid, this time-consuming effort can't be accomplished quickly enough!

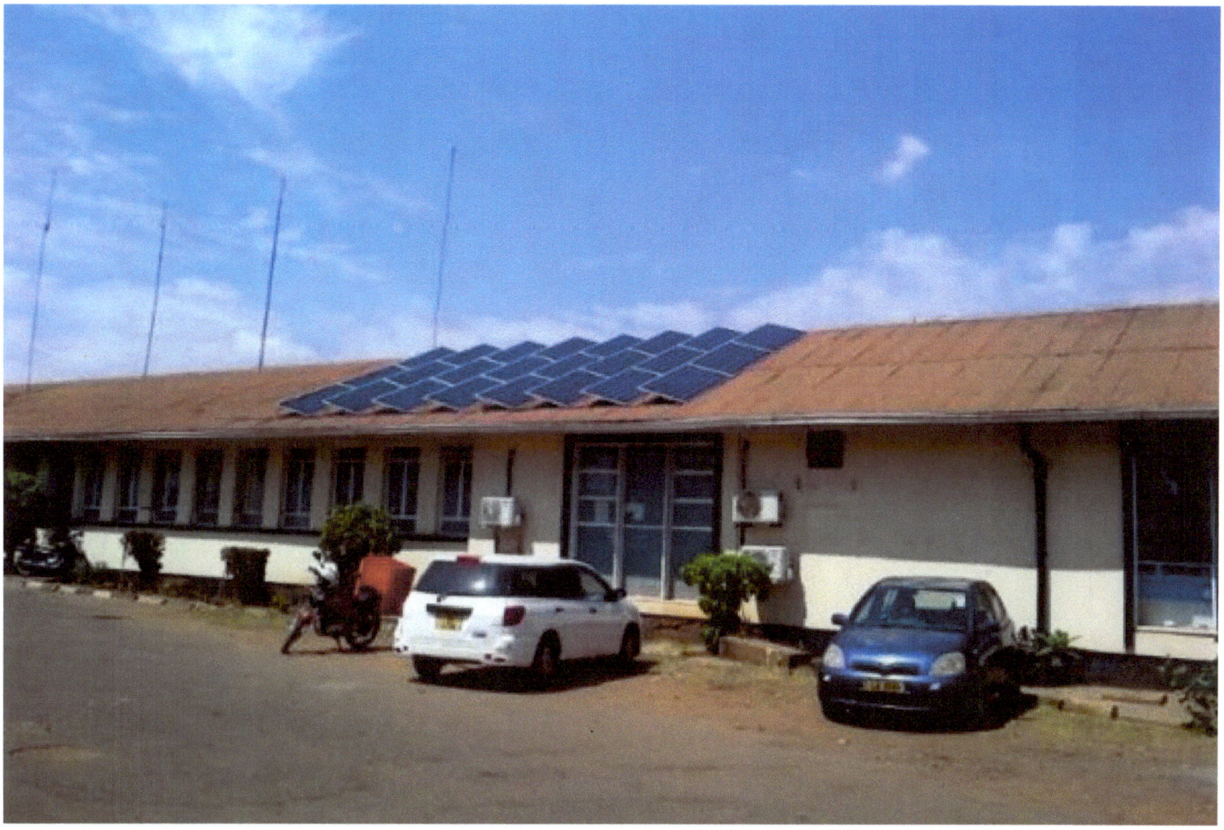

Kasungu District Hospital, solar panels. Photo courtesy of the Nysa Times

Overcrowded hospitals, limited staff, lack of supplies, and blackouts are huge hurdles to the Malawian Healthcare System, but one must first arrive at a hospital to encounter them. Dr. Miriam, a doctor, and teacher at the Malawi College of Health Sciences shared her wish for change, "I'd improve on roads for easy access by ambulances to hospitals and purchase more ambulances."

Long distances to health facilities, which can include crossing rivers and passing through inadequate roads make travel for medical help perilous. Sadly, travel delays during any medical emergency can be fatal.

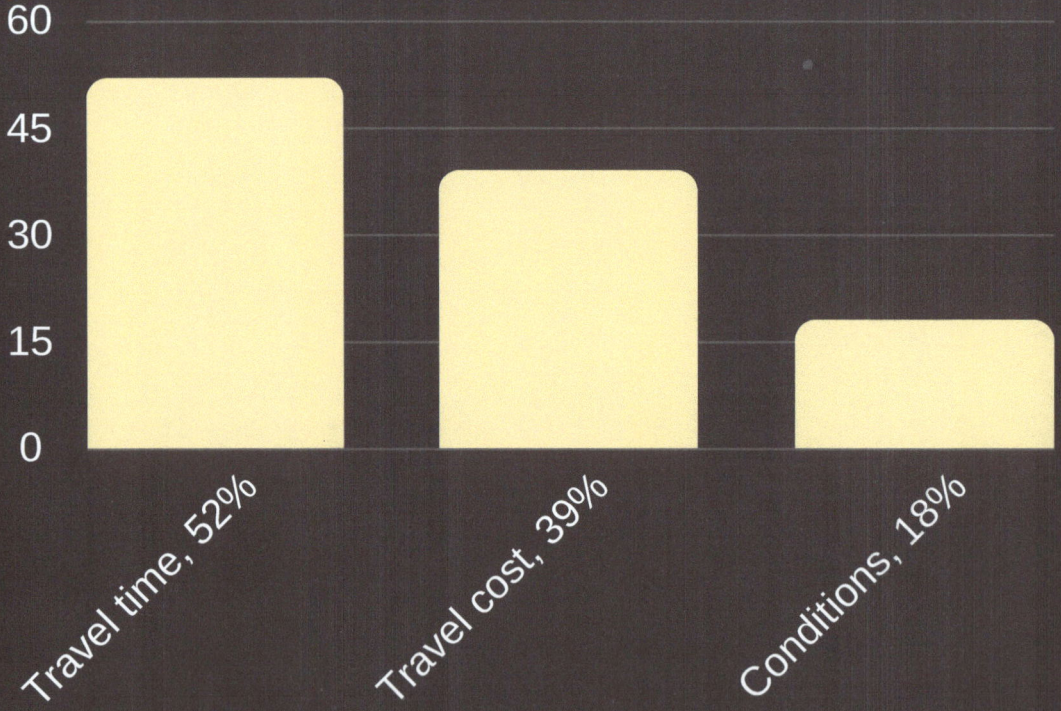
Travel delays in Maternal Deaths in Mangochi

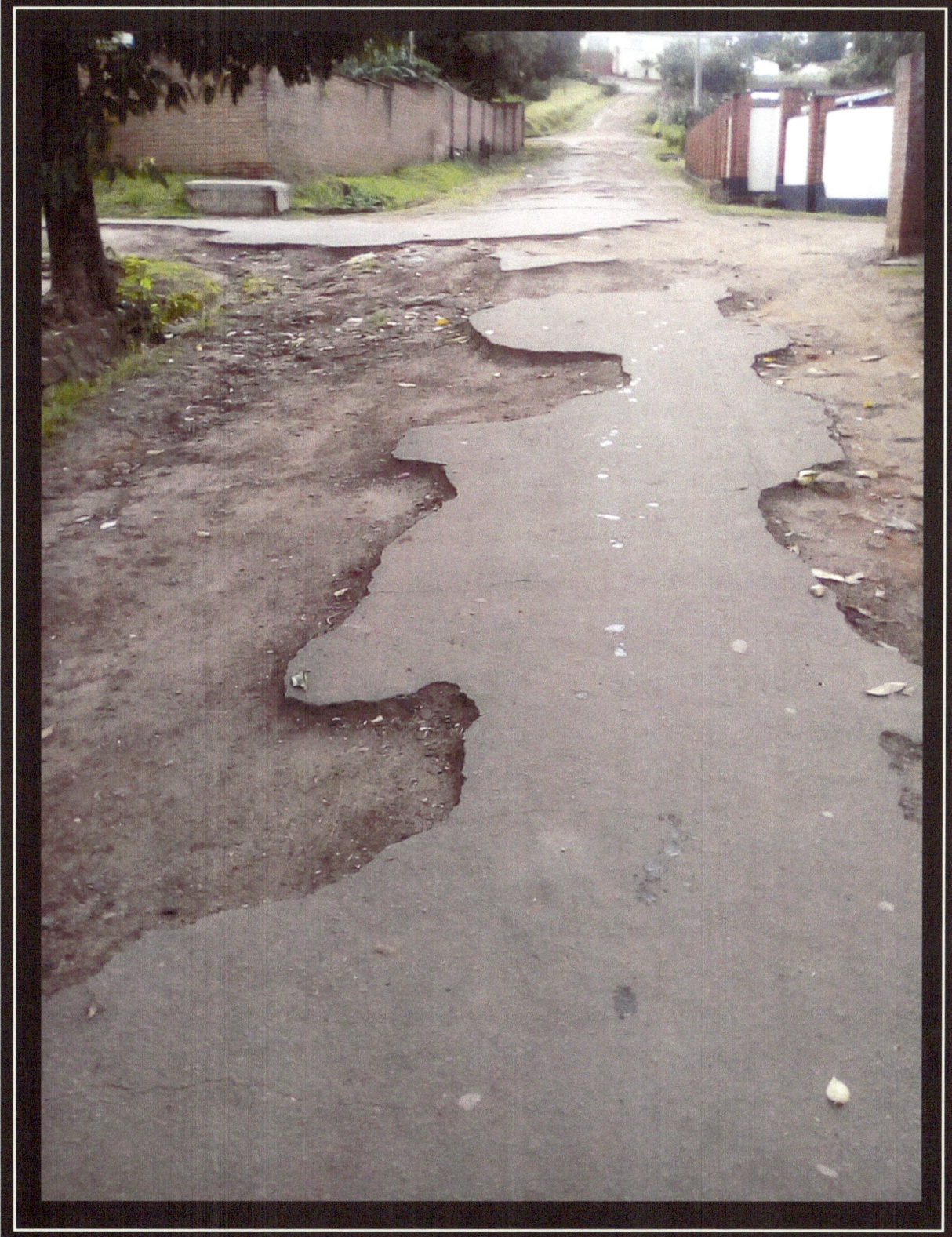

Many women in rural areas find themselves crossing rivers and traveling down un-maintained roads to reach a hospital. Six women in Mangochi used an ox cart to transport them to the hospital and sadly did not return home (Mgawadere, 2017).

Women living in urban areas are closer to healthcare facilities but face the challenge of higher transportation costs. It's estimated that families spent an average of two hours trying to obtain funds for adequate transportation while women labored (Mgawadere, 2017).

Reflections of a New Mom:

"When I found out I was pregnant, I was excited because I would be called a mother. This was my first birth and my fear was the way of giving birth and how I can travel when my time comes. The hospital was not close."

This ambulance was donated by UKAide. Often ambulances serve multiple purposes within a community and wait times can exceed 2 hours.

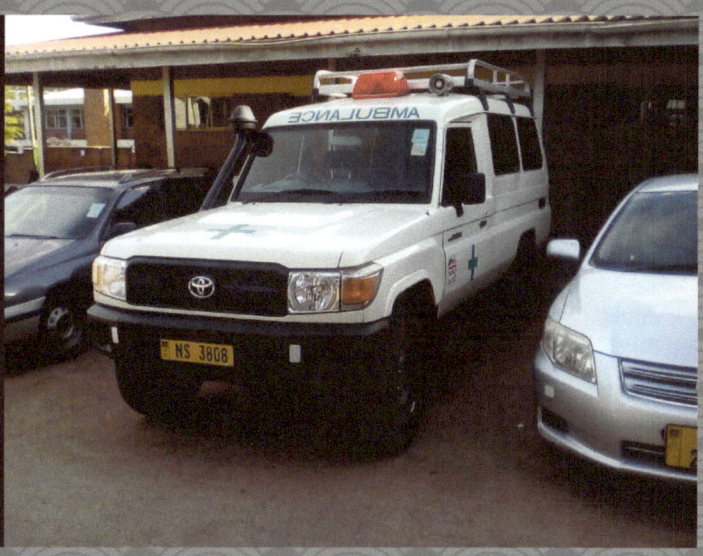

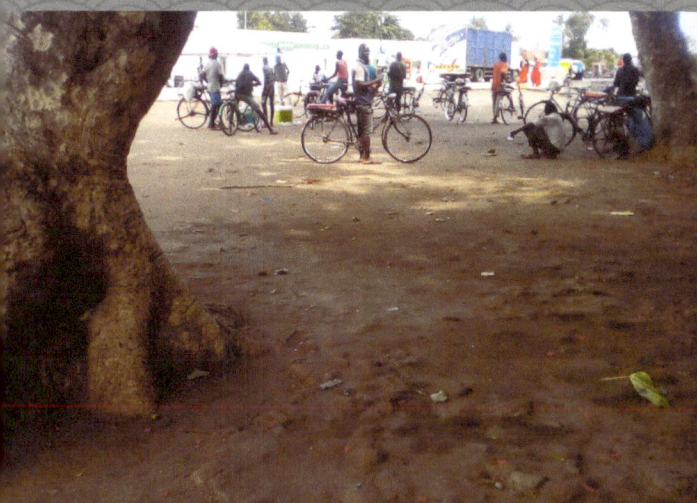

Bicyclists offer transportation to hospitals for approximately $5.

Buses are another way to access hospitals for a woman in urban areas. Bus fare starts at 60 cents.

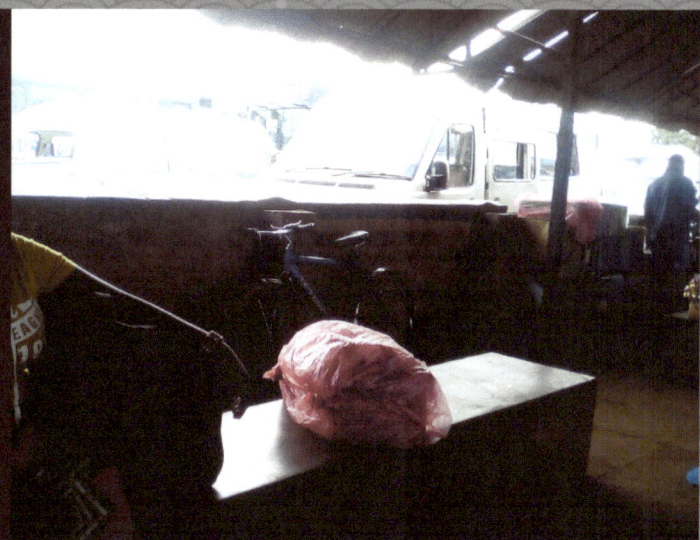

If improving the maternal mortality rates was a simple process, it would have been accomplished long before. Though the problems facing the Malawian Health Care System are mountainous, there are small steps that can have a lifesaving impact. By purchasing this book, you've already taken the first step with us!

Each book sold provides a box of fifty hospital-grade latex gloves to Malawian hospitals in need. In 2018, we believe that no one should die because of a lack of gloves.

To learn about more ways to help and track the progress of this project, please join us at:

EsthersHousePublishing.com/birthinblantyre

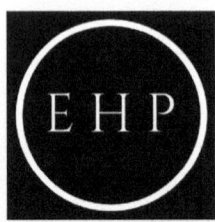

Work Cited:

"Guidelines For Professional Registered Nursing Staffing For Perinatal Units." Association of Women's Health, Obstetric, and Neonatal Nurses, 2010, c.ymcdn.com/sites/www.awhonn.org/resource/download/20150923_084518_19352/SG-910.pdf.

Kane, R.L., Shamliyan, T., Mueller, C., Duval, S., &Wilt, T. (2007). Nursing staffing and quality of patient care (Evidence Report/ Technology Assessment No. 151) Prepared by the Minnesota Evidence-based Practice Center under Contract No. 290-02-0009. AHRQ Publication No. 07-E005. Rockville, MD: Agency for Healthcare Research and Quality.

Meki, Ntchindi. "Space Crisis in Hospitals." The Nation, 10 Feb. 2018, mwnation.com/space-crisis-hospitals/.

Mgawadere, Florence, et al. "Factors associated with maternal mortality in Malawi: application of the three delays model." BMC Pregnancy and Childbirth, vol. 17, no. 1, Dec. 2017, doi:10.1186/s12884-017-1406-5.

Muheya, Green .
 "Malawi public hospitals hit by electricity crisis." Nyasa Times, 8 Nov. 2017, www.nyasatimes.com/malawi-public-hospitals-hit-electricity-crisis-nurses/.

National Statistical Office (NSO) [Malawi] and ICF. 2017. Malawi Demographic and Health Survey 2015-16.
Zomba, Malawi, and Rockville, Maryland, USA. NSO and ICF.

World Health Organization, UNICEF, UNFPA, World Bank, United Nations Population Division. Trends in maternal mortality 1990 to 2015: estimates by the WHO, UNICEF, UNFPA, the World Bank and the United Nations population division. Geneva: World Health Organization; 2015. Available from: http://www.who.int/reproductivehealth/publications/monitoring/maternal-mortality-2013/en/

About the photographer:

Rev. Edward Mikwamba
Rapha Holiness Ministries

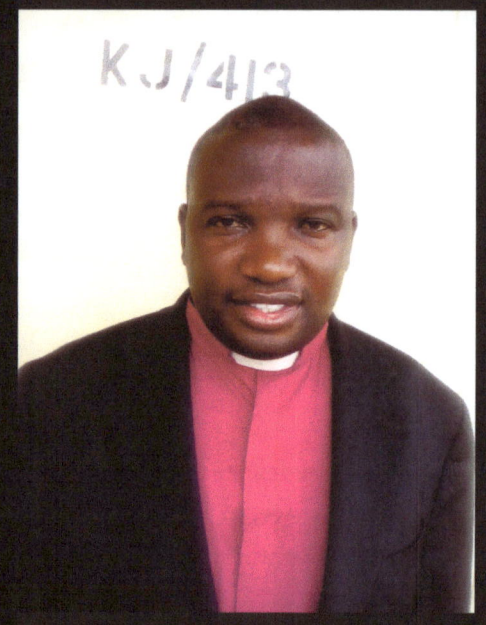

"My goal is to find and fend for the less privileged"

"Before going into full-time ministry I worked for Malawi News and Trans World Radio as a Christian Journalist. I have authored two Books in Chichewa, our native language. One on Stewardship and another on communication.

I like writing and traveling. I was Youth Pastor with Church of the Nazarene for Malawi, Zambia and Zimbabwe for 5 years and traveled to countries training youths. I also studied at the Evangelical Bible college of Malawi.

I am married to Beautiful wife Edna with Children Stephano, Rhoda, Phillip and Step Son Edwin."

A very special thank you to:

Edward Mikwamba
Rapha Holiness Ministry
Martha Yalu
Rose and Robert Mtwuana
Catherine Change
Rosetta Swinton
Nurse Jean
Dr. Miriam
Martha Mtuwana
Princess Mikwamba
and
Re:Birth

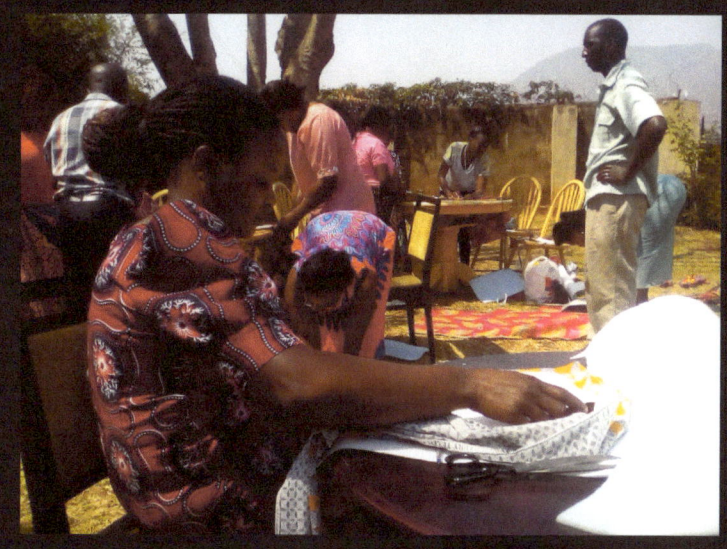

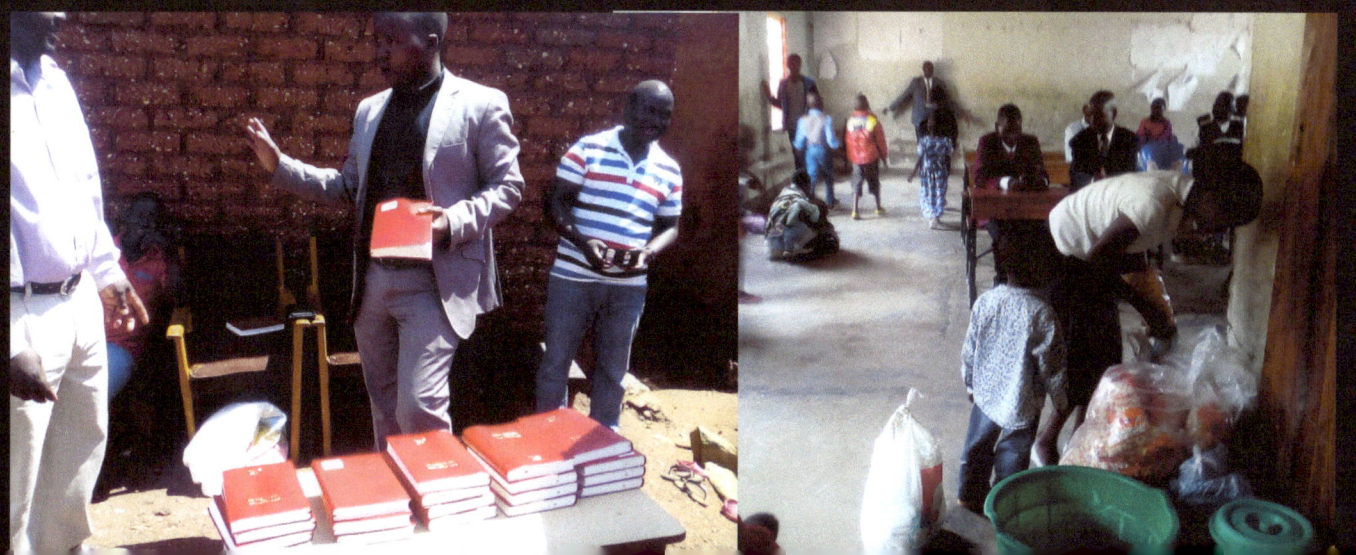

About Esther's House Publishing: Publishing with Purpose

What if every book you picked up served a global purpose? At Esther's House Publishing, we produce unique books for readers of all ages which educate, entertain, and give back to organizations in a powerful way. Through in-house pieces, and custom fundraising books, our books are on a mission and our readers are giving back through each purchase.

Follow the impact of this book at
www.esthershousepublishing.com/birthinblantyre

www.ingramcontent.com/pod-product-compliance
Lightning Source LLC
Chambersburg PA
CBHW051825210526
45473CB00005B/1747